# NCLEX

# Pharmacology: The NCLEX Trainer: Content Review, 100+ Specific Practice Questions & Rationales, and Strategies for Test Success

## Eva Regan

# Contents

publisher.

# Section 1: Introduction

Pharmacology is the branch of medicine concerned with the science of drug action on biological systems. As a licensed nurse, one of your main responsibilities is to administer medication to your clients. When administering medication, whether man-made or natural, a nurse should always know how a medication acts in the body, what the safe administration guidelines for that medication are, as well as understand the risks and implications associated with medication administration. When applying their knowledge of pharmacology, nurses must not only know how to safely administer medication but are at times also required to instruct their client or their client's family on the safe administration of medication. Because of this, it is crucial to have a solid understanding of pharmacology and its application within nursing practice.

For test takers, pharmacology is one of the most difficult topics to master. This is because new medications are constantly emerging and there are already an enormous amount of available medications in common use. It is therefore important to spend enough time reviewing pharmacology in your preparation for the NCLEX. In the exam, you may be presented with a medication that you are not familiar with. In this case you will need to be able to make an educated guess. In this guide, you will be provided with strategies and guidelines that you can apply in order to make an educated guess.

The guide begins with an outline of the topics and key facts that you need to remember for the exam. The list of subtopics can be seen on the contents page. This is all presented with helpful notes, tips, and cautions. In Section 3 of this guide you can apply and test your knowledge with over 100 topic-specific practice questions. All answers to the questions are given with detailed rationales to further your knowledge and understanding of the topic. Smart study strategies are outlined in the penultimate section of this guide - this will put you on a steady path to achieving success on your NCLEX exam!

Remember that ambition is the first step to success. The second step is action – hard work and determination. Purchasing this guide is an indication of your ambition, now it's time to get to work!

Best wishes,

Eva Regan

# Section 2: Pharmacology Study Checklist

## 1. Three Areas of Pharmacology

It's important to remember that pharmacology includes three areas:

**Pharmacokinetics:**

This is the study of how medications are absorbed, metabolized, distributed and excreted by the body.

Pharmacokinetics is particularly relevant when it comes to clients with renal or liver disease or elderly clients who frequently encounter difficulties when it comes to metabolizing and excreting medications.

**Pharmacodynamics:**

This is the study of how medications are used by the body.

**Pharmacotherapeutics:**

This is the study of how the client responds to the drug.

# 2. Pharmacology In Nursing Practice

In nursing practice, nurses are expected to apply their knowledge of pharmacology in order to:

- Recognize common uses, side effects, and adverse effects of their client's medication.
- Meet the learning needs of their client.
- Challenge medication errors.

Test takers need to remember the medication classifications commonly used in medical and surgical settings and their effects on the body:

- **Antacids:** Antacids reduce hydrochloric acid in the stomach. Constipation is a common side effect of calcium- and aluminum-based antacids. Diarrhea is a common side effect of magnesium-based antacids.

- **Anti-infectives:** Anti-infectives are used to treat infections. A common side effect includes GI upset.

- **Antianemics:** Antianemics increase red blood cell production by increasing the amount of haemoglobin in the blood or number of red blood cells. B12, iron, and Epogen (erythropoetin) are all examples of antianemics.

- **Anticholinergics:** Anticholinergics are used to induce dryness in mucous membranes which causes a decrease in oral secretions. Anticholinergics such as atropine are often administered prior to operations.

- **Anticoagulants:** Anticoagulants prevent the coagulation, i.e. clotting of blood. They achieve this by preventing platelet aggregation or by decreasing vitamin K levels and blocking the clotting chain.

- **Anticonvulsants:** Anticonvulsants are used in the treatment of seizure disorder and of bipolar disorder. Phenobarbital, phenytoin (Dilantin), and lorazepam (Ativan) are all medications in this category.

- **Antidiarrheals**: Antidiarrheals reduce water content in the intestinal tract and lower gastric motility. Bloating and gas are common side effects.

- **Antihistamines:** Antihistamines block the release of histamine during allergic reactions. Signs of dry mouth, drowsiness, and sedation are common side effects caused by antihistamines.

- 
- **Antihypertensives:** Antihypertensives lower blood pressure as well as increase blood flow to the myocardium. Orthostatic hypotension is a common side effect. Other side effects may arise which are specific to types of antihypertensive prescribed.

- **Antipyretics:** Antipyretics reduce fever.

- **Bronchodilators:** Bronchodilators dilate large air passages. They are commonly prescribed for clients who suffer from asthma and chronic obstructive lung disease. Tachycardia is a common side effect.

- **Diuretics:** Diuretics decrease the absorption of water and sodium from the loop of Henle (loop diuretics) or inhibit antidiuretic hormone (potassium-sparing diuretics). Hypokalemia is a side effect of non-potassium-sparing diuretics.
- **Laxatives:** Laxatives loosen stools and increase bowel movements. Types of laxatives include cathartics, fiber, lubricants, stimulants, and stool softeners.

- **Miotics:** Miotics onstrict the pupil. Miotics such as pilocarpine HCl are used to treat clients with glaucoma.

-

- **Mydriatics:** Mydriatics dilate the pupils. They are used to treat clients with cataracts.

- **Narcotic analgesics:** Narcotic analgesics are drugs that relieve moderate to severe pain. A common side effect is numbness. They can also induce a state of unconsciousness. Opioids (morphine and codeine), synthetic opioids (meperidine), and NSAIDs (ketorolac) are all medications in this category.

# 3. Administering Medications

The 'Seven Rights' of Administering Medication is a checklist that needs to be memorized by every nursing student and nurse. They include five rights of drug administration and two rights that stem from the Patient's Bill of Rights. The seven rights must be used every time a client is administered a medication by a nurse.

The 'Seven Rights' of Patient Medication include:

4. The Right Medication
5. The Right Patient;
6. The Right Dose;
7. The Right Time;
8. The Right Route;
9. The Right Reason
10. The Right Documentation.

**The Right Medication:** The nurse should check both the generic and trade names with the physician's order in order to ensure that the correct medication is administered. In the case that the client's diagnosis does not match the drug category, the nurse must investigate the ordered medication.

**The Right Patient:** The nurse should take steps to identify the client by checking the identification band and by asking the client to state his name.

**The Right Dose:** The nurse must know common dosages for both adults and children.

**The Right Time:** The nurse is expected administer the medication either 30 minutes before or 30 minutes after the assigned time.

**The Right Route:** The physician orders the prescribed route of administration. This should be followed provided it complies with formulary guidelines.

**The Right Reason / Right to Refuse Treatment:** The client has the right to refuse treatment, which includes medications, if a client refuses medication, the nurse should determine the reasons for refusal.

**The Right Documentation:** The nurse must always document treatment given to the client. Documentation must be done promptly and accurately to ensure that medication administration is not duplicated.

# 4. Time-Released Drugs

Medication that contains one of the abbreviations below are 'time-released drugs.' This means they should under no circumstances be opened, dissolved or crushed before being administered to the client.

- Contin = Continuous action
- CR = Continuous release
- Dur = Duration
- LA = Long acting
- SA = Sustained action
- SR = Sustained release

**Enteric-coated tablets and caplets:** These are medications that are coated with a thick shell. This allows for the medication to be absorbed more slowly and prevents the medication from being absorbed in the upper GI tract.

**Spansules:** These are capsules that contain time-released beads that are released slowly. If the client cannot swallow a time-released medication, then the physician should be notified in order to obtain a different preparation for the client. The nurse should never alter the preparation.

# 5. Drug Schedules

Nurses and nursing students must also know the various drug schedules. This will no doubt crop up in questions relating to safety.

- **Schedule I:** Not currently accepted for medical use and are for research use only (for example, LSD). These are drugs with high potential for abuse.

- **Schedule II:** These drugs have a high potential for abuse and therefore require a written prescription for each refill. Examples of drugs under this schedule narcotics, stimulants and barbiturates for example. No telephone renewals are allowed.

- **Schedule III:** These require a new prescription after six months or five refills. Examples of drugs under this schedule include codeine, steroids, and antidepressants. Can be ordered by telephone.

- **Schedule IV:** These require a new prescription after six months, e.g. benzodiazepines.

- **Schedule V:** These can be dispensed as any other prescription or without prescription (if state law allows). Examples of drugs under this schedule include antidiarrheals and antitussives.

# 6. Pregnancy Categories

One can never say whether it is 100% safe to use a medication on a pregnant client. Because of this, medications are split up into categories of safety by risk level. There are certain categories of medication a pregnant client must avoid and it is important for a nurse to be aware of these categories. Knowledge of these categories is also likely to be tested on the NCLEX exam

- **Category A:** The safest drugs to take during pregnancy. No risk to fetus.

- **Category B:** Insufficient data to use in pregnancy. Studies for fetal effects in animals have found no risks but no adequate studies on pregnant women are available.

- **Category C:** Potential benefits of medication may warrant use of this medication on pregnant women despite potential risks.

- **Category D:** Risk to fetus exists, but potential benefits of the medication could outweigh the probable risks.

- **Category X:** There is positive evidence of human fetal risk. Avoid use of these medications in pregnancy or in those who may become pregnant. Potential risks to the fetus outweigh the potential benefits.

# 7. Herbal Remedies

Although herbals are not considered to be medications by some, they do however have medicinal properties. On the NCLEX exam, herbals are included as a subtopic under pharmacology. The following is a list of the most common herbals used and the necessary guidelines a nurse or nursing student should be aware of.

**Echinacea:**

- Uses: To treat fevers, colds and urinary tract infections.
- Reactions: This herbal can potentially interfere with methotrexate, ketoconazole and immunosuppressive agents.

**Feverfew:**

- Uses: To treat and prevent migraines, arthritis, and fever.
- Reactions: This herbal should not be taken in conjunction with aspirin, NSAIDs, Coumadin, thrombolytics, or antiplatelet medications. This is because it will prolong the bleeding time.

## Ginkgo:

- Uses: This herbal improves memory and can be used to treat depression. Ginkgo also promotes peripheral circulation.
- Reactions: This herbal should not be taken with MAO inhibitors, anticoagulants, or antiplatelets. This is because it increases the bleeding time in clients taking NSAIDs, cephalosporins, and valproic acid. Ginkgo should also be avoided by clients with seizure disorders because it can exacerbate seizure activity.

## Ginseng:

- Uses: Ginseng is used as an anti-inflammatory. This herbal enhances the immune system, improves mental and physical abilities and has estrogen effects.
- Reactions: Ginseng decreases the effects of anticoagulants and NSAIDs. This herbal must be avoided by clients taking corticosteroids. This is because ginseng and corticosteroids when taken in combination can result in extremely high levels of corticosteroids. High doses cause liver problems. Clients with hypertension and bipolar disorder must be cautioned regarding the use of ginseng because it

can interfere with medications used to treat these disorders.

## Kava-kava:

- Uses: Kava-kava is used to treat insomnia as well as mild muscle aches and pains.
- Reactions: This herbal increases the effects of central nervous system (CNS) suppressants and decreases those of levodopa. The use of kava-kava can also increase the effect of MAOIs and cause liver damage.

## Ma Huang:

- Uses: Ma Huang is used for weight loss and to increase energy levels. It is also used to treat asthma and hay fever.
- Reactions: This herbal increases the effect of MAOIs, cardiac glycosides, theophylline, and sympathomimetics.

## St. John's Wort:

- Uses: This herbal is used to treat mild to moderate depression.
- Reactions: St. John's Wort increases adverse CNS effects when used with alcohol or antidepressant medications.

# 8. Understanding and Knowing How to Identify Drugs

Firstly, it is important to understand that drugs have several names:

- **The chemical name:** This is usually a number or letter that is indicative of the chemical makeup of the medication. This name is not of much value to a practicing nurse.
- **The generic name:** This is the name given to the drug by the company that developed it. It is much safer for a nurse to remember this name because the generic name always remains the same.
- **The trade name:** once a drug has been released to the market for around four years, a trade-named medication can be released by another company. While the generic name will stay the same, the trade name will be different.

If you can, it is best to remember both the trade and the generic name of a drug. On the exam, the generic name will be given and the trade name may at times be included for further clarification.

Roughly 80% of generic drugs within the same category have common syllables. Recognizing and identifying these commonalities will significantly help you study for the NCLEX. The following categories in this section are designed to help you recognize these commonalities in the drug names. This will help you to quickly identify a specific drug and thereby their drug category.

1. *Angiotensin-Converting Enzyme (ACE) Inhibitors*
- **Uses:** These Antihypertensives are used in the treatment of both primary and secondary hypertensions.
- **Reactions:** These drugs inhibit conversion of angiotensin I to angiotensin II.
- **Syllable:** PRIL.

You will notice that all the generic names include the syllable 'pril'. If you see the syllable 'pril', this is an indication that the medication is an ACE enzyme inhibitor. Examples include:

Benazepril (Lotensin), lisinopril (Zestril), captopril (Capoten), enalapril (Vasotec), fosinopril (Monopril), moexipril (Univas), quinapril (Acupril), ramipril (Altace). On top of identifying an ACE inhibitor, it is important that you know and remember the potential side effects and adverse reactions of ACE enzyme inhibitors when working with the drug.

## Side effects and adverse reactions associated with ACE inhibitors include:

- Angioedema
- Hacking cough
- Hypotension
- Nausea and/or vomiting
- Rashes

## Nursing considerations to know and use when working with ACE inhibitors:

- Monitor the electrolyte levels
- Monitor the potassium and creatinine levels
- Monitor the vital signs frequently
- Monitor the white blood cell count

2. _Angiotensin Receptor Blockers_
- **Uses:** Angiotensin receptor blockers are used to treat primary or secondary hypertension. These drugs are used to treat clients who complain of coughing that can be linked ot the use of ACE inhibitors.
- **Reactions:** These drugs block vasoconstrictor- and aldosterone-secreting angiotensin II.
- **Syllable:** SARTAN.

When you see the syllable 'sartan', you'll know that the drug is an angiotensin receptor blocker. Examples include:

Candesartan (Altacand), Losartan (Cozaar), Valsartan (Diovan), and Telmisartan (Micardis).

**Side effects and adverse reactions associated with angiotensin receptor blockers include:**

- Cough
- Depression
- Diarrhea
- Dizziness
- Impotence
- Insomnia
- Muscle cramps
- Nausea/vomiting
- Neutropenia

**Nursing interventions to know and use when working with clients that are taking angiotensin receptor blocker agents:**

- Instruct the client to check edema in feet and legs daily.
- Monitor blood pressure.
- Monitor BUN.
- Monitor creatinine.
- Monitor electrolytes.
- Monitor hydration status.

3. *Anticoagulants*
- **Uses:** Anticoagulant drugs are used to treat deep-vein myocardial infarction, pulmonary emboli, thrombosis and thrombolytic disease. These medications are also used after coronary artery bypass surgery and for other conditions, such as those requiring anticoagulation.
- **Reactions:** These drugs thin the blood and are therefore used to treat clotting disorders.
- **Syllable:** PARIN.

When you see the syllable 'parin', you'll know that the drug is a anticoagulant. Examples include: Dalteparin sodium (Fragmin), Enoxaparin Sodium (Lovenox), and Heparin Sodium (Hepalean).

**Side effects and adverse reactions associated with anticoagulant drugs include:**

- Alopecia
- Bleeding
- Dermatitis
- Diarrhea
- Fever
- Hematuria
- Pruritus
- Stomatitis

**Nursing interventions to know and use when working**

**with clients that are taking anticoagulant agents:**

- Check blood studies (hematocrit and occult blood in stool) every three months
- Monitor for signs of bleeding
- Monitor for signs of infection
- Monitor platelet count
- Perform a PTT check on clients taking **Heparin Sodium** (Hepalean) to evaluate the bleeding time (therapeutic levels are 1.5–2.0 times the control)
- No specific bleeding time is done for **Enoxaparin Sodium** (Lovenox), but platelet levels must be checked for thrombocytopenia

4. *Anti-Infectives (Aminoglycosides)*
- **Uses:** These drugs are used to either kill an infectious agent or inhibit it from spreading.
- **Reactions:** Anti-infective drugs interfere with the protein synthesis of bacteria, thereby causing the bacteria to die. Anti-infectives are active against some gram-positive organisms and against most aerobic gram-negative bacteria.
- **Note:** Anti-infectives are often used in the treatment of super-infections, e.g. methicillin-resistant staphylococcus aureus (MRSA). The symptoms of clients with MRSA include: cough, diarrhea, fever, malaise, pain, perineal itching, redness, stomatitis and swelling.

- **Syllable:** CIN or MYCIN.

Anti-infectives include bactericidals and bacteriostatics. These drugs end with the syllable 'cin' and many of them end in 'mycin.' Examples include: Gentamicin (Garamycin, Alcomicin, Genoptic), kanamycin (Kantrex), neomycin (Mycifradin), streptomycin (Streptomycin), tobramycin (Tobrex, Nebcin), amikacin (Amikin).

## Side effects and adverse reactions associated with anti-infectives include:

- Blood dyscrasias
- Hypotension
- Nephrotoxicity
- Ototoxicity
- Rash
- Seizures

## Nursing interventions to know and use when working with clients that are taking anti-infectives:

- Obtain history of allergies
- Instruct the client to report any chances in renal function, i.e. urinary elimination, or in hearing. (This is because these drugs can be toxic to the auditory nerve and to the kidney)
- Monitor for therapeutic levels
- Monitor for signs of nephrotoxicity
- Monitor for signs of ototoxicity

- Monitor a patent IV site
- Monitor intake and output
- Monitor peak and through levels
- Monitor vital signs during intravenous infusion

5. *Antivirals*
- **Uses:** Antivirals are used for their antiviral properties. Clients that suffer from AIDS are often treated with either one or a combination of antiviral. Antiviral drugs are also used in the treatment of HSV-1 and HSV-2, chickenpox, shingles, fever blisters, encephalitis, cytomegalovirus (CMV), and respiratory syncytial virus (RSV).
- **Reactions:** Antivirals inhibit enzymes with a virus, thereby inhibiting viral growth.
- **Syllable:** VIR.

When you see the syllable 'vir', you'll know that the drug is an antiviral. Examples include: Acyclovir (Zovirax), Abacavir (Ziagen), Cidofovir (Vistide), Indinavir (Crixivan), Ritonavir (Norvir), and Saquinovir (Invirase, Fortovase).

**Side effects and adverse reactions associated with antivirals include:**

- Diarrhea
- Nausea

- Oliguria
- Proteinuria
- Vaginitis
- Vomiting
- Central nervous side effects are also possible although these are less common:
    - Tremors
    - Confusion
    - Seizures
    - Severe/sudden anemia

**Nursing interventions to know and use when working with clients that are taking antiviral drugs:**

- Be watchful for signs of infection
- Instruct the client to report any signs of a rash as this can be indicative of an allergic reaction
- Monitor bowel pattern before and during treatment
- Monitor liver profile

Monitor the creatinine level frequently

6. *Benzodiazepines (Anticonvulsants/Antianxiety) drugs*
- **Uses:** Benzodiazepines are used for their anti-anxiety or anti-convulsant effects, e.g. to reduce anxiety, to induce relaxation, to treat or prevent seizures and panic disorders, among other things.
- **Syllable:** PAM, PATE, or LAM.

When trying to identify benzodiazepines, it is useful to remember that while some contain the syllable 'pam', others contain 'pate' or 'lam'. All benzodiazepines however will contain 'azo' or 'aze'. Examples include Clonazepam (Klonopin), diazepam (Valium), chlordiazepoxide (Librium), lorazepam (Ativan), flurazepam (Dalmane)

**Side effects and adverse reactions associated with benzodiazepines include:**

- Ataxia
- Bradycardia
- Constipation
- Depression
- Diplopia
- Drowsiness
- Hypotension
- Incontinence
- Lethargy
- Nausea/vomiting
- Nystagmus
- Rash
- Respiratory depression
- Restlessness
- Slurred speech
- Urinary retention
- Urticaria

**Nursing interventions to know and use when working**

## with benzodiazepines:

- Monitor respirations
- Monitor liver function
- Monitor kidney function
- Monitor bone marrow function
- Monitor for signs of chemical abuse

7. *Beta Adrenergic Blockers*
- **Uses:** These drugs help lower blood pressure, pulse rate, and cardiac output. Beta adrenergic blockers are also used in the treatment of migraines and other vascular headaches. Certain preparations of this drug can also be used in the treatment of glaucoma and to prevent myocardial infarctions.
- **Reactions:** Beta adrenergic blockers act by blocking the sympathetic vasomotor response.
- **Syllable:** OLOL.

When you see the syllable 'olol', you'll know that the drug is a beta blocker. Examples include Acebutolol (Monitan, Rhotral, Sectral), Atenolol (Tenormin, Apo-Atenol, Nova-Atenol), Carvedilol (Coerg), Esmolol (Brevibloc) and Toprol-XL (Metoprolol). On top of being able to identify beta adrenergic blockers, nurses and nurse students must also know the potential side effects and adverse effects.

**Side effects and adverse reactions associated with beta**

**adrenergic blockers include:**

- Bradycardia
- Diarrhea
- Nausea and/or vimiting
- Orthostatic hypertension
- May mask hypoglycemic symptoms

**Nursing interventions to know and use when working with clients that are taking beta adrenergic blockers:**

- Teach the client to:
  - o Taper off the medication
  - o Rise slowly
  - o Report bradycardia, dizziness, confusion, depression or any signs of fever
- Monitor the client's blood pressure, heart rate, and rhythm
- Monitor the client for changes in lab values (BUN, creatinine, protein) that indicate nephrotic syndrome
- Monitor the client for signs of edema. The nurse must assess lung sounds for rhonchi and rales.

8. *Cholesterol-Lowering Agents*
- **Uses:** Cholesterol-Lowering Agents are use to reduce cholesterol and triglyceride levels. These drugs are also used decrease the potential for cardiovascular disease and to

- **Note:** Cholesterol-lowering drugs should not be taken with grapefruit juice. They should be taken at night and the client must have undergone liver studies prior to taking cholesterol-lowering agents to determine the presence of liver disease.
- **Syllable:** VASTATIN.
- **Caution:** Do not confuse with 'statin' drugs that are used for their antifungal effects, such as Nystatin.

When you see the syllable 'vastatin', you'll know that the drug is a cholesterol-lowering agent. Examples include: Atorvastatin (Lipitor), fluvastatin (Lescol), lovastatin (Mevacor), pravastatin (Pravachol), simvastatin (Zocar), rosuvastatin (Crestor).

## Side effects and adverse reactions associated with cholesterol-lowering drugs include:

- Alopecia
- Dyspepsia
- Headache
- Liver dysfunction
- Myalgia (muscle weakness)
- Rash

## Nursing interventions to know and use when working with clients that are taking cholesterol-lowering agents:

- Include a diet low in cholesterol and fat

- Instruct the client to report any unexplained muscle soreness or weakness and cola-colored urine to the physician
- Monitor cholesterol levels
- Monitor for muscle weakness and pain
- Monitor liver profile
- Monitor renal function

9. *Glucocorticoids*

- **Uses:** Glucocorticoids are used to decrease inflammatory responses to allergies and inflammatory diseases, to reduce the possibility of organ plant rejection, and to treat conditions that require suppression of the immune system. These drugs are also used in the treatment of Addison's disease, chronic obstructive pulmonary disease, and immune disorders.

- **Reactions:** Glucocorticoids have anti-allergenic, anti-inflammatory, and anti-stress effects.

- **Note:** Glucocorticoid drugs can cause Cushing's syndrome. Symptoms include buffalo hump, edema, elevated blood glucose levels, hirsutism, moon faces, purple straie, and weight gain.

- **Syllable:** SONE or CORT.

When you see the syllable 'sone' or 'cort', you'll know that the drug is a glucocorticoid. Examples include: Prednisolone (Delta-Cortef, Prednisol, Prednisolone), prednisone (Apo-

Prednisone, Deltasone, Meticorten, Orasone, Panasol-S), betamethasone (Celestone, Selestoject, Betnesol), dexamethasone (Decadron, Deronil, Dexon, Mymethasone, Dalalone), cortisone (Cortone), hydrocortisone (Cortef, Hydrocortone Phosphate, Cortifoam), methylprednisolone (Solu-cortef, Depo-Medrol, Depopred, Medrol, Rep-Pred), triamcinolone (Amcort, Aristocort, Atolone, Kenalog, Triamolone).

## Side effects and adverse reactions associated with glucocorticoid drugs include:

- Acne
- Bruising
- Depression
- Depression
- Diarrhea
- Ecchymosis
- Flushing
- Hemorrhage
- Hypertension
- Hypomania
- Insomnia
- Leukocytosis
- Osteoporosis
- Petechiae
- Poor wound healing
- Sweating

## Nursing interventions to know and use when working with clients that are taking glucocorticoid drugs:

- Monitor blood pressure
- Monitor for signs of infection
- Monitor glucose levels
- Weigh the client on a daily basis

10. *Histamine 2 Antagonists*
- **Uses:** Histamine 2 antagonist drugs are used to decrease acid production and to treat acid reflux, gastric ulcers, and GERD.
- **Reactions:** These agents inhibit gastric acids by inhibiting histamine 2 release in the gastric parietal cells.
- **Syllable:** TIDINE.

When you see the syllable 'tidine', you'll know that the drug is a histamine 2 antagonist. Examples include: Cimetidine (Tagamet), Famotidine (Pepcid), Nizatidine (Axid), and Rantidine (Zantac).

**Side effects and adverse reactions associated with histamine 2 antagonists include:**

**Confusion**

- Agranulocytosis
- Alopecia
- Bradycardia/tachycardia
- Diarrhea

- Galactorrhea
- Gynecomastia
- Psychosis
- Rash
- Seizures

**Nursing interventions to know and use when working with clients that are taking histamine 2 antagonist drugs:**

- Administer the drugs with meals
- Cimetidine can be prescribed in one large dose at bedtime
- If the client is taking antacids as well as histamine 2 antagonists, make sure the client takes antacids one hour before or after taking these medications
- Monitor the blood urea nitrogen levels
- Sucralfate reduces the effects of histamine 2 receptor blockers

11. _Phenothiazines (Antipsychotic/Antiemetic) drugs_
- **Uses:** Phenotiazines are used as antiemetics, neuroleptics or major tranquilizers. These drugs are used in the treatment of psychosis in clients with schizophrenia. Certain phenothiazine drugs, e.g. Phenergan (promethazine) and Compazine (prochlorperzine), are used to treat nausea and vomiting.
- **Note:** Phenotiazines are irritating to the tissue. Because of this, Z-track method should be used to

administer this drug by intramuscular injection. A client who is allergic to this a phenothiazine drug is likely to be allergic to all of them. A client who experiences an allergic reaction, extrapyramidal effects or any more severe reactions needs to be given **Congentin** (benztropine mesylate) or **Benadryl** (hdiphenhydramine hydrochloride).

- **Syllable:** ZINE.

When you see the syllable 'ZINE', you'll know that the drug is a phenothiazine. Examples include: Chlopromazine (Thorazine), prochlorperazine (Compazine), trifluoperazine (Stelazine), promethazine (Phenergan), hydroxyzine (Vistaril), fluphenazine (Prolixin).

**Side effects and adverse reactions associated with phenothiazines include:**

- Agranulocytosis
- Drowsiness
- Dry mouth
- Extrapyramidal effects
- Neuroleptic malignant syndrome
- Orthostatic hypotension
- Photosensitivity
- Sedation

**Nursing interventions to know and use when working with clients that are taking phenothiazines:**

- Be cautious: liquid forms of Fluphenazine (Prolixin) should not be mixed with any beverage containing caffeine, tannates, or pectin due to physical incompatibility
- Monitor liver enzymes
- Monitor renal function
- Protect the client from overexposure to the sun
- Protect the drug from light

## 12. *Proton Pump Inhibitors*

- **Uses:** Proton pump inhibitors are used to treat indigestion, esophagitis, gastric ulcers, and GERD.
- **Reactions:** These inhibitors inhibit the hydrogen/potassium ATPase enzyme system, thereby suppressing gastric secretion.
- **Syllable:** PRAZOLE.

When you see the syllable 'prazole', you'll know that the drug is a proton pump inhibitor. Examples include: Esomeprazole (Nexium), Lansoprazole (Prevacid), Pantoprazole (Protonix), and Rabeprazole (AciPhex).

**Side effects and adverse reactions associated with proton pump inhibitors include:**

- Diarrhea
- Flatulence

- Headache
- Hyperglycemia
- Insomnia
- Rash

**Nursing interventions to know and use when working with clients that are taking proton pump inhibitors:**

- Instruct the client to always take the medication prior to meals
- Monitor liver function
- Use a filter when administering IV pantoprazole – don't crush pantoprazole (Protonix)

To pass the NCLEX, you will need to learn the specific classification of a drug. Remember that learning these classifications will make studying for the pharmacology significantly easier - this is because medications within a certain category share the same commonalities.

When revising for the NCLEX, it is therefore crucial to remember:

- The specific classification of a medication, its actions inside the body, and all associated side effects and adverse effects
- How to safely administer a medication within that specific classification

# 9.  Other Useful Drug Identification Clues:

Below are some other clues helpers that can assist you in identifying drug types:

- **Caine** = Anesthetics (Lidocaine)
- **Cal** = Calciums (Calcimar)
- **Ceph or cef** = Cephalosporins (Cefatazime)
- **Cillin** = Penicillins (Ampicillin)
- **Cycline** = tetracycline (Tetracycline) (Note that Tetracycline should never be given to a pregnant woman or small children)
- **Done** = Opioids (Methodone)
- **Mab** = Monoclonal antibodies (Palivazumab)
- **Phylline** = Bronchodilators (Aminophylline)
- **Stigmine** = Cholinergics (Phyostigmine)

*Looking at the similarities and commonalities between medications will help you to identify a certain type of drug, know their side effects and the relevant nursing interventions. This will also help you manage and divide the substantial knowledge that you need to successfully pass the test.*

*I encourage you to review this section often to ensure you remember all essential facts and information. Do not worry if you don't feel entirely confident yet - start testing yourself on realistic practice questions which you can find in the next section. Go over any questions you get incorrect, working out why, and then improve your knowledge in that specific area.*

# Section 3: Practice Questions and Rationales

1. While acquiring information about the current medication use of the client, the client tells the nurse that he takes the herbal supplement ginkgo to improve mental alertness. The nurse should inform the client to:

   a. Avoid any exposure to the sun whilst using ginkgo.

   b. Buy only brands with FDA approval.

   c. Increase daily intake of vitamin E.

   d. Report signs of bleeding or bruising or to the doctor.

**Answer D is correct.** Ginkgo interacts with many different medications to increase the risk of bleeding. Because of this, bruising or bleeding should be reported to the doctor. Answer A is incorrect, because photosensitivity is not a side effect of ginkgo. The FDA does not regulate herbals and natural products, and therefore Answer B is also incorrect. Lastly, the client does not need to take additional vitamin E, answer C is therefore also incorrect.

2. The client has a prescription for a calcium carbonate compound in order to neutralize stomach acid. The

**nurse should assess the client for:**

    a. Diarrhea

    b. Constipation

    c. Hyperphosphatemia

    d. Hypomagnesemia

**Answer B is correct.** A client using calcium preparations will frequently develop constipation. Answers B, C, and D do not apply in this scenario.

3. **Which of the following medications are category X medications and should therefore not be taken by the client during pregnancy?**

    a. Cefozolin
    b. Devonex
    c. Levothyroxine
    d. Menocycline
    e. Tazorac

**Answers B, D, and E are correct.** Devonex, Minocycline, and Tazorac and are all medications under category X and should therefore not be given during pregnancy because they are teratagenic.

4. **Your client is taking alendronate sodium (Fosamax). Which instruction should you give to your client?**

   a. Remain in an upright position for 30 minutes after taking this medication
   b. Take the medication while lying down
   c. Force fluids while taking this medication
   d. Take the medication together with estrogen

**Answer A is correct.** This drug causes gastric reflux, so the client should remain upright and take it with only water. Alendronate sodium is a drug used in the treatment of osteoporosis. Alendronate sodium should not be taken while lying down and should not be taken in conjunction with another medication or with estrogen.
Notice: there is a clue in the name of the drug: *fosa*, as in fossils. All the drugs in this category contain the syllable *dronate*.

5. **A client is discharged with a prescription for Evista (raloxifene HCl). The nuse should inform the client of which of the following is a side effect of this drug?**

   a. Urinary frequency
   b. Leg cramps
   c. Hot flashes
   d. Cold extremities

**Answer C is correct.** Evista is a drug used in the treatment of osteoporosis. The medication has an agonist effect, which binds with estrogen and which can cause hot flashes. The medication does not cause any of the other symptoms and answers A,B, and D are therefore incorrect.

Notice: The E in Evista stands for estrogen. This medication is in the same category as the chemotherapeutic agent tamoxifene (Novaldex) which is used for breast cancer.

6. **The client, an elderly diabetic, is scheduled for a cardiac catheterization. The client has been taking metformin (Glucophage). The nurse should instruct the client to:**

    a. Take the medication with only water prior to the exam
    b. Take the medication as usual prior to the exam
    c. Limit protein intake prior to the exam
    d. Discontinue the medication prior to the exam

**Answer D is correct.** This is because Glucophage can cause renal problems. The dye used in cardiac catheterizations is likewise detrimental to the kidneys. After the cardiac catheterizations or until renal function returns, the client may be placed on sliding scale insulin for 48 hours.

Note that B and D are opposites. B is incorrect because the client should stop taking the medication prior to the exam. Answer A is incorrect because taking Glucophage with water is not necessary. And Answer C is likewise incorrect because limiting protein intake prior to the exam has no correlation to the medication.

Notice: The syllable 'phage' (as seen in the syllable 'phage') means eating.

7. **The client is taking furosemide (Lasix). Which of the following laboratory results should be of concern to the nurse?**

    a. Sodium level of 140
    b. Potassium level of 2.5
    c. Glucose level of 110
    d. Calcium level of 8

**Answer B is correct.** This is because Furosemide (Lasix) is a loop diuretic.

Notice: Most loop diuretics end in the syllable 'ide'.

8. **A client who has just undergone an exploratory laparotomy is admitted to the recovery room. Which of the following medication should be kept nearby?**

    a. Diphenhydramine (Benadryl)
    b. Flumazenil (Romazicon)
    c. Naloxone hydrochloride (Narcan)
    d. Nitroprusside (Nipride)

**Answer C is correct.** Answer C is correct because Narcan is the antidote to narcotics. During the postoperative period, narcotics are given to the client. Answer A is also incorrect because Benadryl is an antihistamine. Answer B is incorrect because Romazicon is the antidote for the benzodiazepines. Answer D is incorrect because Nipride is used to lower blood pressure.

9.  **The client with renal failure has a subscription for erythropoietin (Epogen) which is to be given subcutaneously. The nurse should instruct the client to report which of the following symptoms?**

    a. Decreased urination
    b. Itching
    c. Severe headache
    d. Slight nausea

**Answer C is correct.** This is because severe headache can indicate impending seizure activity. It should therefore be immediately reported. Answer A and C are incorrect because a client with renal failure already suffers from itching and decreased urination. Answer D is incorrect because slight nausea is expected when beginning the therapy.

10. **A four-year-old client with cystic fibrosis has an order for Viokase pancreatic enzymes to prevent**

**malabsorption. The pancreatic enzyme should be administered:**

    a. On an empty stomach

    b. One hour before meals

    c. Two hours after meals

    d. With each meal and snack

**Answer D is correct.** Viokase is a pancreatic enzyme used to facilitate digestion. The enzyme should therefore be given with meals and snacks. Viokase works well in foods such as applesauce. Answers A, B, and C are all incorrect.

11. **A 20-year-old client has an order for tetracycline. While teaching the client how to take the medicine, the nurse is told that the client is currently also using Ortho-Novum, an oral contraceptive pill. The nurse should inform the client that:**

    a. Antibiotics can decrease the effectiveness of oral contraceptives. Because of this, the client should use different type of birth control.

    b. Nausea often results from taking oral contraceptives and antibiotics.

    c. The oral contraceptives will decrease the effectiveness of the tetracycline.

d. Toxicity can result when taking these two medications together.

**Answer A is correct.** Taking both antibiotics and oral contraceptives at the same time decreases the effectiveness of the oral contraceptives. The client should therefore be advised to take use a different type of birth control.

12. **The nurse is visiting a home health client with osteoporosis who has a new prescription for alendronate (Fosamax). Which instruction should be included in the teaching plan?**

a. Avoid rapid movements after taking Fosamax.

b. Don't take any other medications for 30 minutes after taking the Fosamax.

c. Rest in bed for at least half an hour after taking the medication.

d. Take the medication with water only and remain upright for at least 30 minutes after taking the medication.

**Answer D is correct.** Fosamax should be taken with water only. The client should also remain upright for at least 30 minutes after taking the medication. Answer C is the opposite of Answer D and is therefore incorrect. Answers A and B are not applicable to taking Fosamax and are therefore also incorrect.

13. **The client diagnosed with multiple myeloma has a subscription for cyclophosphamide (Cytoxan). The nurse should instruct the client to:**

    a. "Drink at least eight large glasses of water a day."
    b. "Immediately report nausea to the doctor."
    c. "Increase the fiber intake in your diet."
    d. "Walk for at least 30 minutes a day to prevent calcium loss."

**Answer A is correct.** The medication can cause hemorrhagic cystitis and because of this, the client should drink at least eight glasses of water a day. Answers B is incorrect as nausea often occurs with chemotherapy. Answers C and D are both not necessary and are therefore incorrect.

14. **The nurse is guiding the mother through the treatment for enterobiasis. Which instruction should be included in the teaching plan?**

    a. Intravenous antibiotic therapy will be ordered.
    b. Medication therapy will continue for one year.
    c. The entire family should be treated.
    d. Treatment is not recommended for children under the age of 10 years.

**Answer C is correct.** Pinworms (enterobiasis) is treated using Vermox (mebendazole) or Antiminth (pyrantel pamoate). To make sure no worms remain, it is important that the entire family is treated. The family should get tested again after two weeks. Answers A, B and D do not apply and are therefore incorrect.

15. **Lidocaine is a medication frequently prescribed for the client experiencing:**

    a. Atrial tachycardia

    b. Heart block

    c. Ventricular brachycardia

    d. Ventricular tachycardia

**Answer D is correct.** Lidocaine increases the electric stimulation threshold of the ventricles without depressing the force of ventricular contractions, thereby exerting an antiarrhythmic effect. The medication is therefore used in the treatment of ventricular tachycardia. Answer A is incorrect because Lidocaine is not used for atrial arrhythmias. Answers B and C are incorrect because Lidocaine slows down the heart rate and it is therefore not used for brachycardia or heart block.

**16. The client is scheduled for a Tensilon test to check for Myasthenia Gravis. Which of the following drugs should be kept available during the test?**

    a. Atropine sulfate

    b. Promethazine

    c. Prostigmin

    d. Furosemide

**Answer A is correct.** This is because atropine sulfate is the antidote for Tensilon and is therefore used to treat cholenergic crises. Answers B, C, and D are all incorrect. Answer B is incorrect because Promethazine is an antiemetic anti-anxiety medication. Answer C is incorrect because Prostigmin is utilized to treat myasthenia gravis. Answer D is incorrect as Furosemide is a diuretic.

**17. Which of the following should be used in the treatment of iron toxicity?**

    a. Desferal (deferoxamine)

    b. Digibind (digoxin immune Fab)

    c. Narcan (naloxone)

    d. Zinecard (dexrazoxane)

**Answer A is correct.** Desferal is used to treat iron toxicity.

Answer B is incorrect because Digibind is used to treat dioxin toxicity. Answer C is incorrect because Narcan is used to treat narcotic overdose. Answer D is incorrect because is utilized to treat doxorubicin toxicity. Answers B, C, and D are all antidotes for other medications.

**18. The physician has prescribed Amoxil (amoxicillin) 500mg capsules for a client with esophageal varices. The nurse can best care for the client by:**

    a. Administering the medication with an antacid

    b. Giving the client the medication as ordered

    c. Providing extra water with the medication

    d. Requesting the medication in an alternative form an alternate form of the medication

**Answer D is correct.** The client with esophageal varices could potentially develop spontaneous bleeding from the mechanical irritation caused by taking capsules. Because of this, the nurse should request an alternate form of the medication, for example a suspension. Answer A is incorrect because Amoxil should not be given with milk or antacids. Answer B is incorrect because this would not be in the best interest of the client. Answer C is incorrect because providing extra water is not a good means of preventing bleeding.

19. The physician has prescribed Dilantin (phenytoin) 100mg for a client with generalized tonic clonic seizures to be administered intravenously. The nurse should administer the medication:

    a. Rapidly with an IV push

    b. Through a small vein

    c. With IV dextrose

    d. Slowly over 2–3 minutes

**Answer D is correct.** Dilantin should be administered slowly – no more than 50mg per minute as cardiac arrhythmias can otherwise occur. Answer A is incorrect because the drug must be administered slowly. Answers B and C are also incorrect. Dextrose solutions cause the medication to crystallize in the line and the medication should therefore be administered through a large vein in order to prevent "purple glove" syndrome.

20. The nurse finds that the respiratory rate of a post-operative client has dropped from 14 breaths per minute to 6 breaths per minute. The nurse gives the client Narcan (naloxone) as per standing order. After Narcan has been administered, the nurse should assess the client for:

    a. Projectile vomiting

    b. Pupillary changes

c. Sudden, intense pain

d. Wheezing respirations

**Answer C is correct.** The medication Narcan is a narcotic antagonist that blocks the effects of the client's pain medication. Because of this, the client will experience sudden, intense pain. Answers A, B, and D are incorrect because they do not relate to the condition of the client in relation to the administration of Narcan.

21. **A client with congestive heart failure has been maintained with digoxin (Lanoxin). Which of the following indicates that the drug is having a desired effect?**

   a. Improved appetite

   b. Increased pedal edema

   c. Increased urinary output

   d. Stabilized weight

**Answer C is correct.** The medication slows and strengthens the contraction of the heart. An increase in urinary output therefore shows that Lanoxin is having a desired effect by eliminating excess fluid from the body. Answers A, B, and D are all incorrect. Answer A is incorrect because it is not related to the medication. Answer B is incorrect because pedal edema would decrease and not increase. Answer D is incorrect because the client's weight would decrease.

**22. The physician has prescribed the medication Basaljel (aluminum carbonate gel) for a client with recurrent indigestion. The nurse should inform the client of the side effects that come from using the medication, which include:**

    a. Confusion

    b. Constipation

    c. Diarrhea

    d. Urinary retention

**Answer B is correct.** Constipation is a common side effect of Basaljel, which is an antacid that contains aluminum. Answers A, C, and D are all incorrect as they are not common side effects of the medication.

**23. A client in labor has an order for Demerol (meperidine) 75 mg. IM which is to be administered 10 minutes before delivery. The nurse should:**

    a. Administer the medication as ordered

    b. Administer the medication IM during the delivery to prevent pain from the episiotomy

    c. Question the order

d. Wait until the client is placed on the delivery table then give the medication

**Answer C is correct.** Giving a narcotic to a pregnant client close to the time of delivery can result in respiratory depression in the newborn. Because of this, the nurse should question the order. Answers A, B, and D are all incorrect for the very same reason.

24. **The physician has ordered Synthroid (levothyroxine) for a client with myxedema. Which statement shows that the client understands the nurse's instruction regarding the medication?**

   a. "I will check my heart rate before taking the medication."

   b. "I will take the medication every morning after breakfast."

   c. "If I develop gastric upset, I will stop taking the medication."

   d. "If I experience any visual disturbance, I will report this to my doctor."

**Answer A is correct.** The client should be instructed and taught to the check their heart rate before taking the medication. This is because Synthroid (levothyroxine) increases metabolic rate and cardiac output and adverse reactions to the medication include tachycardia and dysrhythmias. Answer B is incorrect because the client does not have to take the medication after breakfast. Answer C is incorrect as the medication should not be stopped if the client develops gastric upset. Answer D is also incorrect because it has no relation to the medication.

25. **A client who has recently been diagnosed with diabetes has started receiving Precose (acarbose). The nurse should instruct the client to take the medication:**

    a. 1 hour before meals

    b. 30 minutes after meals

    c. Every day at bedtime

    d. With the first bite of a meal

**Answer D is correct.** The medication should be taken with the first bite of a meal. Answers A, B and C are all incorrect.

26. **A 6-year-old client is being treated for an acute attack of asthma using racemic epinephrine (epinephrine hydrochloride) nebulizer stat. Which of the following indicates an adverse effect of this medication?**

    a. Excitability

    b. Heart rate 150

c. Nausea

d. Tremors

**Answer B is correct.** This is because hypertension and tachycardia are both adverse effects of epinephrine. Answers A, C, and D are all incorrect in this case as these are expected side effects of racemic epinephrine.

27. **The client is being treated with intravenous Vancomycin for MRSA. The nurse notices redness of the neck and chest of the client. Place in ordered sequence the actions that the nurse should take:**

   a. Administer Benadryl as ordered

   b. Call the doctor

   c. Stop the IV infusion of Vancomycin

   d. Take the vital signs

**The correct order is C, D, B, A.**

28. **A client with leukemia has been receiving oral prednisolone (Prednisone). Which of the following is an expected side effect of the prolonged use of prednisolone?**

   a. Decreased appetite

   b. Hirsutism

c. Integumentary bronzing

d. Weight loss

**Answer B is correct.** Hirsutism, or facial hair, is a side effect of cortisone therapy. Answers A, C, and D are all incorrect. These are symptoms of Addison's disease.

29. **The physician has prescribed DDAVP (desmopressin acetate) for a client with diabetes insipidus. Which of the following is an indication that the medication is having a desired effect?**

    a. A decline in the client's urinary output

    b. An increase in the client's activity level

    c. The client has an improved appetite

    d. The client's morning blood sugar was 120mg/dL

**Answer A is correct.** A declined in urinary output shows that the drug is having its desired effects. This is because excessive production of dilute urine is a characteristic of diabetes insipidus. Answers B and C are incorrect as they are not related to the question. Answer D is incorrect as it refers to diabetes mellitus.

30. **A 15-year-old client with cystic acne has an order for Accutane (isotretinoin). Prior to starting the medication, which lab work is needed?**

   a. Clean-catch urinalysis

   b. Liver profile

   c. Complete blood count

   d. Thyroid function test

**Answer B is correct.** The medication Accutane consists of concentrated vitamin A, which is a fat-soluble vitamin. A liver panel is needed as fat-soluble vitamins can potentially become hepatotoxic. Answers A, C, and D are incorrect as they do not relate to therapy with Accutane.

31. **A post-operative client has a prescription for Demerol (meperidine) 75mg and Phenergan (promethazine) 25mg IM every 3–4 hours as required to counter pain. When taken in combination, the two medications produce:**

   a. A Excitatory effect

   b. A Synergistic effect

   c. An Agonist effect

   d. An Antagonist effect

**Answer B is correct.** The two medications when taken in combination produce a synergistic effect, that is, an effect that is greater than that of either drug used alone. Answer A is incorrect because the two drugs combined would have a depressing effect, and not an excitatory effect. Answer C is incorrect because agonist effects are similar to those produced by chemicals normally present in the body. Answer D is incorrect because antagonist effects are those in which the actions of the medications oppose one another.

32. **Prior to giving a client's morning dose of Lanoxin (digoxin), the nurse checks the apical pulse rate. She finds a rate of 54. The appropriate nursing intervention in this instance is to:**

   a. Administer the medication and monitor the heart rate

   b. Record the pulse rate and administer the medication

   c. Withhold the medication and notify the doctor

   d. Withhold the medication until the heart rate increases

**Answer C is correct.** The appropriate nursing intervention in this scenario is to best provide for the client's safety by withholding the medication and notify the doctor. Answers A, B, and D are incorrect.

33. **A client with schizophrenia has started receiving Zyprexa (olanzapine). Three weeks later, the client develops severe muscle rigidity and elevated temperature. The nurse should give priority to which of the following interventions:**

    a. Administering prescribed anti-Parkinsonian medication

    b. Ordering a CBC and CPK

    c. Transferring the client to a medical unit

    d. Withholding all morning medications

**Answer A is correct.** Severe muscle rigidity and elevated temperature are symptoms that suggest that the client is experiencing an adverse reaction to the medication known as as neuroleptic malignant syndrome. Answers B, C, and D are incorrect as they are not appropriate interventions.

34. **A child with cystic fibrosis is receiving inhalation therapy with Pulmozyme (dornase alfa). Which of the following is a side effect of the medication?**

    a. Brittle nails

    b. Hair loss

    c. Sore throat

    d. Weight gain

**Answer C is correct.** Side effects of Pulmozyme include hoarseness, laryngitis, sore throat. Answers A, B, and D are incorrect because they are not associated with Pulmozyme.

35. **A client who has been maintained with Dilantin (phenytoin) for tonic-clonic seizures is preparing for discharge. Which of the following should be included in the client's discharge care plan?**

    a. A high-carbohydrate diet must be avoided

    b. Regularly scheduled blood work will be needed

    c. The medication can cause dental staining

    d. The medication can cause problems with drowsiness

**Answer B is correct.** The client will need regularly scheduled blood work because agranulocytosis and aplastic anemia are potential adverse side effects of Dilantin. Answer A is incorrect because the drug does not interfere with the metabolism of carbohydrates. Answer C is incorrect because Dilantin does not cause dental staining. Answer D is incorrect because Dilantn does not cause any problems related to drowsiness.

36. **The doctor has prescribed Cortone (cortisone) for a client with systemic lupus erythematosis. Which instruction should be given to the client?**

a. Report changes in appetite and weight to the doctor

b. Schedule a time to take the influenza vaccine every year

c. Take the medication 30 minutes before meals

d. Wear sunglasses to prevent cataracts

**Answer B is correct.** This is because a client who is receiving steroid medication should also receive an annual influenza vaccine. Answer A is incorrect because weight gain and an increased appetite are both expected side effects of steroid medication. Answer C is incorrect because the medication should be taken with meals. Answer D is incorrect because wearing sunglasses does not prevent cataracts in the client taking Cortone.

37. **The physician has prescribed Stadol (butorphanol) for a post-operative client. The nurse knows that the medication is having its desired effect if the client:**

a. Has an increased urinary output

b. Is asleep for 30 minutes after the injection

c. Reports that he/she is feeling less nauseated

d. States that he/she is still feeling hungry

**Answer B is correct.** The medication reduces the perception of pain, which allows the post-operative client to rest. Answers A and D are incorrect as these are not affected by the medication. Answer C is incorrect because, although pain relief can reduce symptoms of nausea, it is not a desired effect of the Stadol.

38. **A client is hospitalized with hepatitis A. Which of the client's regular medications is contraindicated due to the current illness?**

   a. Lipitor (atorvastatin)

   b. Premarin (conjugated estrogens)

   c. Prilosec (omeprazole)

   d. Synthroid (levothyroxine)

**Answer A is correct.** Lipid-lowering agents are contraindicated in the client with active liver disease. Answers B, C, and D are incorrect as they are not contraindicated in the client with active liver disease.

39. **A client with diabetes mellitus has a prescription for Glucotrol XL (glipizide). The client should be instructed to take the medication:**

   a. With breakfast

   b. Before lunch

c. After dinner

d. At bedtime

**Answer A is correct.** Glucotrol XL is to be taken once a day with breakfast. Answers B and C are incorrect because the client would hypoglycemia later in the day or evening. Answer D is incorrect because the client would also develop hypoglycemia while sleeping.

40. **The physician has prescribed Vancocin (vancomycin) 500mg IV every six hours for a client with MRSA. The medication should be administered in the following manner:**

    a. IV push

    b. Over 15 minutes

    c. Over 30 minutes

    d. Over 60 minutes

**Answer D is correct.** The medication should be given very slowly so as to prevent "redman" syndrome. Answer A is incorrect because Vancomycin is not given IV push. Answers B and C are also incorrect because the medication should be administered at a slower rate.

41. **The nurse calculates the amount of an antibiotic for injection to be administered to an infant. The**

amount of medication to be given is 1.25mL. Which of the following is the correct way to administer the antibiotic?

  a. Administer the medication in one injection in the dorsogluteal muscle

  b. Administer the medication in one injection in the ventrogluteal muscle

  c. Divide the amount in two injections and administer one in the ventrogluteal muscle and one in the vastus lateralis muscle

  d. Divide the amount into two injections and administer in each vastus lateralis muscle

**Answer D is correct.** This is because no more than 1mL should be administered in the vastus lateralis of an infant. Answers A, B, and C are all incorrect because the other two muscles, the dorsogluteal and ventrogluteal muscles, are not used for injections in the infant.

42. **An 65-year-old client with glaucoma is scheduled for a cholecystectomy. Which of the following drug prescriptions should the nurse question?**

  a. Atropine (atropine)
  b. Demerol (meperidine)
  c. Phenergan (promethazine)
  d. Tagamet (cimetadine)

**Answer A is correct.** This is because Atropine increases intraocular pressure and is contraindicated in the client with glaucoma. Answers B, C, and D are incorrect as they are not contraindicated in the client with glaucoma.

43. **The physician has prescribed Dilantin (phenytoin) for a client with generalized seizures. When planning the client's care, the nurse should:**

    a. Check the client's pulse prior to administering the medication

    b. Give the medication 30 minutes before meals

    c. Maintain strict intake and output

    d. Provide oral hygiene and gum care at every shift

**Answer D is correct.** The nurse should provide oral hygiene and gum care at every shift because Gingival hyperplasia is a side effect of Dilantin. Answers A, B, and C are incorrect because they do not apply to the medication.

44. **The physician has ordered Cognex (tacrine) for a client with dementia. The nurse should monitor the client for potential adverse reactions, which include:**

    a. Hypoglycemia

b. Jaundice

c. Tinnitus

d. Urinary retention

**Answer B is correct.** The nurse should monitor the client for any symptoms of jaundice. This is because drug-induced hepatitis is an adverse reaction associated to Cognex. Answers A, C, and D are incorrect because these are not among the adverse reactions that can be linked to the medication.

45. **A client exhibiting serum cholesterol of 275mg/dL is placed on rosuvastatin (Crestor). Which instruction should a nurse give to a client using rosuvastatin (Crestor)?**

a. Allow 6 months for the drug to take effect

b. Report any signs of insomnia

c. Report any signs of muscle weakness to the doctor

d. Take the medication with fruit juice

**Answer C is correct.** Crestor is an antilipidemic drug. A client using Crestor must therefore report any signs of muscle weakness as these may be symptomatic of rhabdomyolysis. Answer A is incorrect because the drug takes effect in the first month of starting therapy. Answer B is incorrect because it is unrelated to Crestor. Answer D is also incorrect because mixing the medication with fruit juice, particularly grapefruit, can decrease its effectiveness. Crestor should always be taken with water.

46. **The physician prescribes lisinopril (Zestril) and furosemide (Lasix) to be administered concomitantly to the client with hypertension. The appropriate nursing intervention is to:**

   a. Administer both medications

   b. Administer the medications separately

   c. Contact the pharmacy

   d. Question the order

**Answer A is correct.** Zestril is an ACE inhibitor and Lasix is a diuretic for hypertension. ACE inhibitors are frequently given with diuretics and the nurse should therefore administer both medications. Answers B, C, and D are all incorrect. There is no need to administer the medications separately, to question the order, or contact the pharmacy.

47. **The client with varicella will most likely have a prescription for which category of medication?**

   a. Antibiotics

   b. Anticoagulants

c. Antipyretics

d. Antivirals

**Answer D is correct.** Varicella (chicken pox) is a herpes virus which is best treated with antiviral medications. Answer A and B are both incorrect because the client is not treated with antibiotics or anticoagulants. Answer C is also incorrect because even though the client may have a fever before the chicken pox appear, the temperature will usually go down.

48. **A client with urinary tract infection has a prescription for Pyridium (phenazopyridine hydrochloride). The nurse should inform that client that the medication may:**

a. Cause changes in taste

b. Cause diarrhea

c. Cause mental confusion

d. Turn her urine orange or red

**Answer D is correct.** A nurse should teach clients taking Pyridium that the medication will change the color of her urine. The medication, if taken in large doses, can also result in sclera and pale or yellowed skin. Answers A, B, and C are incorrect as diarrhea, mental confusion or changes in taste are not side effects of the medication.

**49. A client who has recently undergone a heart transplant is started on medication to prevent organ rejection. Which of the below drug categories prevent the formation of antibodies against the new organ?**

    a. Analgesics
    b. Antibiotics
    c. Antivirals
    d. Immunosuppressants

**Answer D is correct.** Immunosuppressants are utilized to prevent the formation of antibodies. Answers A, B, and C are incorrect because analgesics, antibiotics, and antivirals are not used to prevent antibody production.

**50. A physician has ordered streptokinase for a client. Before administering the medication, the nurse should check the client for:**

    a. A history of alcohol abuse

    b. A history of streptococcal infections

    c. Allergies to pineapples and bananas

    d. Prior therapy with phenytoin

**Answer B is correct.** This is because clients with a history of streptococcal infections could have antibodies that make streptokinase ineffective. Answers A, C, and D are incorrect. There is no reason to assess the client for a history of alcohol abuse, allergies to pineapples or bananas, and there is also no correlation to the use of phenytoin and streptokinase.

51. **The nurse has received a pre-op order to administer Valium (diazepam) 10mg and Phenergan (promethazine) 25mg. The correct process of administering these medications is to:**

    a. Question the order because they the two medications cannot be given at the same time

    b. Administer the Valium first and to wait five minutes before injecting the Phenergan

    c. Administer the medications separately

    d. Administer both medications together in one syringe

**Answer C is correct.** Valium is an anti-anxiety drug and Phenergan is an antiemetic. The medications should be administered separately but can be given to the client at the same time. Answer A is incorrect because the two medications can be given to the same client. Answer B is incorrect as there is no need to wait to inject the second medication. Answer D is incorrect because Valium should not be given in same syringe with other medications.

**52. The physician has ordered Cobex (cyanocobalamin) for a client following a gastric resection. Which finding indicates that the medication is having its intended effect?**

    a. Platelet count of 250,000 cu. mm

    b. Neutrophil count of 4500 cu mm

    c. Hgb of 14.2 g/dL

    d. Eeosinophil count of 200 cu mm

**Answer C is correct.** The medication Cobex is an injectable form of vitamin B12 or cyanocobalamin. A lab finding showing an increase in Hgb levels shows that the medication is effective. Answers A, B, and D are incorrect as they are not indicative of the effectiveness of the medication.

**53. A client with paranoid schizophrenia has a prescription for Thorazine (chlorpromazine) 400mg orally twice daily. Which of the following symptoms should immediately be reported to the physician?**

    a. Lethargy, slurred speech, thirst

    b. Fever, sore throat, weakness

    c. Fatigue, drowsiness, photosensitivity

d. Dry mouth, constipation, blurred vision

**Answer B is correct.** Any symptoms of fever, sore throat, and weakness should be reported immediately. Agranulocytosis is a potential adverse effect of Thorazine, which renders the client vulnerable to overwhelming infection. Answers A, C, and D are expected side effects and there is therefore no need to notify the physician immediately.

54. **The doctor has prescribed an infusion of Osmitrol (mannitol) for a client with increased intracranial pressure. Which of the following findings indicates the direct effectiveness of the drug?**

    a. An increased urinary output

    b. An increased pupil size

    c. An increased pulse rate

    d. A decreased diastolic blood pressure

**Answer A is correct.** Osmitrol (mannitol) is an osmotic diuretic, which inhibits reabsorption of sodium and water. An increased urinary output is therefore a direct indication of the effectiveness of the drug. Answers B, C, and D are incorrect as they do not relate to the effectiveness of the drug.

55. The client with a urinary tract infection has an order for Gantrisin (sulfasoxazole) 1gm in divided doses. The nurse should administer the medication:

    a. With meals or a snack
    b. 30 minutes before meals
    c. 30 minutes after meals
    d. At bedtime

**Answer B is correct.** To enhance absorption, Sulfa drugs, including Gantrisin, should be administered 30 minutes before meals. Answer A is incorrect because the drug should be administered prior to meals. Answer C is incorrect because the medication should always be given on an empty stomach. Answer D is incorrect as the medication should be administered in divided doses throughout the course of the day.

56. The mother of a child with chickenpox is inquiring whether there is a medication that can help reduce the course of chickenpox. Which of the following medications can be used to speed up healing of the lesions and thereby shorten the duration of fever and itching?

    a. Periactin (cyproheptadine)

    b. Varivax (varicella vaccine)

    c. VZIG (varicella-zoster immune globulin)

d. Zovirax (acyclovir)

**Answer D is correct.** Zovirax shortens the course of chickenpox, but the American Academy of Pediatrics does not recommend it for healthy children because of the cost. Answer A is incorrect because Periactin is an antihistamine that is used to control itching that results from chickenpox. Answer B is incorrect because Varivax is the vaccine that is used to prevent chickenpox. Answer C is also incorrect as VZIG is the immune globulin that is given to those who have become exposed to chicken pox.

57. **The physician has ordered Chloromycetin (chloramphenicol) for a client with bacterial meningitis. The nurse should pay particular attention to the following lab report:**

    a. Complete blood count

    b. Serum creatinine

    c. Serum sodium

    d. Urine specific gravity

**Answer A is correct.** The nurse should monitor the client's complete blood count most carefully. This is because aplastic anemia is an adverse side effect of chloramphenico. Answers B, C, and D are not directly affected by the medication and are therefore incorrect. Nevertheless, these should be noted down by the nurse.

58. **A client admitted for treatment of bacterial pneumonia has a prescription for intravenous ampicillin. Which specimen should the nurse obtain before administering the medication?**

    a. Complete blood count

    b. Routine urinalysis

    c. Serum electrolytes

    d. Sputum for culture and sensitivity

**Answer D is correct.** The nurse should obtain a sputum specimen for culture and sensitivity before administering the antibiotic in order to check whether the organism is sensitive to the prescribed medication. A, B, and C are all incorrect as a routine urinalysis, complete blood count, and serum electrolytes can be obtained after the therapy has commenced.

59. **The client with angina has an order for nitroglycerin sublingual tablets. The nurse should instruct the client to take the medication:**

    a. After engaging in light exercise

    b. As soon as the client notices signs of chest pain

c. At bedtime to prevent nocturnal angina

d. Every four hours to prevent chest pain

**Answer B is correct.** The client should take the medication as soon as he notices chest pain or discomfort. Answer A is incorrect because the tablets should be taken before engaging in activity. Any strenuous activity should be avoided. Answer C is incorrect because the drugs do not prevent nocturnal angina. Answer D is incorrect because the tablets should be taken when the pain occurs and not according to a regular schedule.

60. **The client is maintained on Lugol's solution prior to a thyroidectomy. The nurse should instruct the client to:**

    a. Take the solution at bedtime

    b. Take the medication with juice

    c. Report changes in appetite

    d. Avoid sunshine while taking the medication

**Answer B is correct.** Lugol's solution is a soluble solution of potassium iodine and because of its bitter taste, it should be given with juice. Answer A is incorrect. Answer C and D are both unnecessary and therefore also incorrect.

61. **A client is to receive Dilantin (phenytoin) via a nasogastric (NG) tube. When administering the drug, the nurse should:**

   a. Administer the medication, flush with 5mL of water, and clamp the NG tube

   b. Flush the NG tube with 2–4mL of water before administering the medication

   c. Flush the NG tube with 2–4oz of water before and after giving the medication

   d. Flush the NG tube with 5mL of normal saline and give the medication

**Answer C is correct.** When administering the medication, the nurse should flush the NG tube twice with 2–4oz of water, that is, before and after giving the medication. Answers A and B are incorrect because insufficient amounts of water are used in both options. Answer D is incorrect because saline should not be used to flush the NG tube.

62. **A client with pneumocystis carinii has an order for Pentam (pentamidine) IV. While receiving the medication, the nurse should carefully monitor the client's:**

   a. Blood pressure

   b. Heart rate

   c. Respirations

d. Temperature

**Answer A is correct.** This is because hypotension is a severe toxic side effect of pentamidine. Answers B, C, and D are incorrect as they are unrelated.

63. **A client in labor has received epidural anesthesia with Marcaine (bupivacaine). Epidural anesthesia produces vasodilation which results in a decrease in blood pressure. To reverse the hypotension caused by epidural anesthesia, the nurse should have which medication nearby?**

   a. Adrenalin (epinephrine)

   b. Dobutrex (dobutamine)

   c. Narcan (naloxone)

   d. Romazicon (flumazenil)

**Answer A is correct.** The nurse should make sure to have adrenalin available to reverse hypotension. Answer B is incorrect because Dobutrex is an adrenergic which increases cardiac output. Answer C is incorrect because Nracan is a narcotic antagonist. Answer D is likewise incorrect because Romazicon is a benzodiazepine antagonist.

**64.** Four clients are to receive medication. Which client should the nurse prioritise?

    a. The client with abdominal surgery receiving Phenergan (promethazine) IM every four hours PRN for nausea and vomiting

    b. The client with an apical pulse of 72 receiving Lanoxin (digoxin) PO daily

    c. The client with labored respirations receiving a stat dose of IV Lasix (furosemide)

    d. The client with pneumonia receiving Polycillin (ampicillin) IVPB every six hours

**Answer C is correct.** The client receiving a stat dose of IV Lasix should be first to receive his medication. Answers A, B, and D are incorrect because these are regularly scheduled medications for clients whose conditions are more stable.

**65. The physician has ordered an injection of morphine for a client with post-operative pain. Before giving the medication, the nurse should check the client's:**

    a. Blood pressure

    b. Heart rate

    c. Respirations

    d. Temperature

**Answer C is correct.** It is absolutely essential for the nurse to assess the client's respirations. This is because Morphine is an opiate and can therefore severely depress the client's respirations. Answers A, B, and D are incorrect.

66. **A client with AIDS tells the nurse that she regularly takes echinacea to boost her immune system. The nurse should inform the client that:**

    a. Herbals can interfere with the action of antiviral medication

    b. Herbals have been shown to decrease the viral load

    c. Supplements appear to prevent replication of the virus

    d. Supplements have proven effective in prolonging life

**Answer A is correct.** The nurse should advise the client to discuss the use of herbals with his doctor because herbal remedies such as echinacea can interfere with the action of antiviral medications. Answer B is incorrect as it has not been shown that herbals can reduce the viral load. Answer C is incorrect because herbals do not prevent replication of the virus. Answer D is incorrect because it has not been shown that herbals can prolong life.

67. **The physician has ordered Activase (alteplase) for a client admitted with a myocardial infarction. Which of the following is a desired effect of Activase?**

    a. An increased tissue oxygenation

    b. The destruction of the clot

    c. The prevention of congestive heart failure

    d. The stabilization of the clot

**Answer B is correct.** The desired effect of Activase, a thrombolytic agent, is to destroy the clot. Answer A is incorrect because increased oxygenation is not a direct result of the medication. Answer C is incorrect because Axtivase does not prevent congestive heart failure. Answer D is incorrect because the medication does not stabilize the clot.

68. **A client informs the nurse that she takes St. John's wort (hypericum perforatum) three times a day to counter mild depression. The nurse should advise the client that:**

    a. It is safe to use the herbal with other antidepressants

    b. She should avoid eating aged cheese

    c. Skin reactions increase with the use of sunscreen

d. The herbal St. John's wort seldom rarely depression

**Answer B is correct.** The herbal St. John's wort has properties similar to those of monoamine oxidase inhibitors (MAOI). Therefore, eating foods high in tryramine such as aged cheese, chocolate, salami, and liver can result in a hypertensive crisis. Answer A is incorrect because the herbal should not be used in combination with MAOI antidepressants. Answer C is incorrect because use of a sunscreen prevents skin reactions to sun exposure. Answer D is likewise incorrect because St. John's wort can relieve mild to moderate depression.

69. **A client with chronic pain is being treated with opioid administration via epidural route. Which medication should be kept nearby and available due to a possible complication of this pain relief procedure?**

    a. Diphenhydramine (Benadryl)

    b. Ketorolac (Toradol)

    c. Naloxone (Narcan)

    d. Promethazine (Phenergan)

**Answer C is correct.** Naloxene should be kept nearby as an antagonist for these medications. This is because Rrspiratory depression can occur from the administration of opioids.

Answers A, B, and D are not necessarily incorrect as they might also be needed, but respiratory depression is the most important and most sever problem that could occur. Benadryl and Phenergan may however be used to treat itching and nausea. Toradol, which is classified as an NSAID, could be used for its anti-inflammatory properties.

70. **The nurse is checking the medication history of a client who was admitted for surgery in the morning. Which long-term medication in the client's history would be most important to report to the doctor?**

    a. Docusate (Colace)

    b. Lisinopril (Zestril)

    c. Oscal D

    d. Prednisone

**Answer D is correct.** The nurse should definitely report usage of prednisone. This is because a sudden withdrawal of steroids could potentially lead to a collapse of the cardiovascular system. Answer A, B, and C are incorrect as these are not so relevant in the maintenance of the steroids. Colace is a stool softener, Zestril is an ACE inhibitor used as an antihypertensive, and Oscal D is a calcium and vitamin agent.

**71. A nurse is working in an endoscopy recovery area. To provide conscious sedation, many of the clients are given midazolam (Versed). Which drug should always be available as an antidote for Versed?**

a. Diazepam (Valium)

b. Florinef (Fludrocortisone)

c. Flumazenil (Romazicon)

d. Naloxone (Narcan)

**Answer C is correct.** Romazicon, a benzodiazepine, is the antidote for Versed, which is used as an antianxiety drug and for conscious sedation. Answers A, B, and D are incorrect as these medications are not used antagonists for Versed.

**72. A client with asthma has a prescription to start an aminophylline IV infusion. Which of the following is essential for the nurse to safely administer the medication?**

a. Cover to prevent exposure of solution to light

b. IV infusion device

c. IV inline filter

d. Large bore intravenous catheter

**Answer B is correct.** An infusion device should be used to regulate Aminophylline, thereby preventing improper infusion rates. Answers A, C, and D are incorrect as they are not necessary for administration of this medication.

73. **A client with osteoporosis is being discharged on alendronate (Fosamax). Which statement would indicate a need for further teaching?**

    a. "After taking Fosamax, I should remain in an upright position for 30 minutes."

    b. "I should not have any food with this medication."

    c. "I should take Fosamax orally with water."

    d. "I should take the medication immediately every night before bedtime."

**Answer D is correct.** Fosamax should be taken in the morning before taking any other medications and before having food. The medication should be taken with water as the only liquid. Statement D is therefore incorrect and is a sign that further teaching is required. All other answers (A, B, and C) are correct administrations.

74. **A client has an order for Demerol 75mg and atropine 0.4mg IM as a preoperative medication. The Demerol vial contains 50mg/mL, and atropine is**

available 0.4mg/mL. The nurse should administer how much medication in total?

a. 1.0mL

b. 1.7mLs

c. 2.5mLs

d. 3.0 mLs

**Answer C is correct.** The calculated dosage of Atropine is 1.0mL, and the calculated dosage of Demerol is 1.5mL, which comes to a total of 2.5mL. Answers A, B, and D are all incorrect calculations.

75. The nurse is discharging a client with asthma with a prescription for zafirlukast (Accolate). Which statement by the client would indicate a need for further teaching?

a. "I should take this medication when eating."

b. "If I'm already having an asthma attack, this drug will not stop it."

c. "My doctor might order liver tests while I'm on this drug."

d. "Should I experience any flu-like symptoms, I should report this to my doctor."

**Answer A is correct.** the medication should be taken either one hour before or two hours after meals. This is to prevent slow absorption of the drug. Statement A is therefore incorrect and is a sign that further teaching is required. Answers B, C, and D are all correct statements.

76. **A physician has prescribed haloperidol (Haldol) for a client with advanced Alzheimer's disease. Which of the following symptoms suggests that the client is experiencing side effects from this drug?**

   a. Cough

   b. Diarrhea

   c. Pitting edema

   d. Tremors

**Answer D is correct.** When taking Haldol, tremors are an extrapyramidal side effect that can occur. Answers A, B, and C are all incorrect and are not side or adverse effects of the medication.

77. **A client with Alzheimer's disease has an order for donepezil (Aricept). Which information should the nurse always include in the teaching plan for a client who is placed on Aricept?**

   a. "If a dose is skipped, take two the next time."

b. "Rise slowly because the medicine can cause dizziness."

c. "Take the medication with meals."

d. "The pill can cause your heart rate to increase."

**Answer B is correct.** Dizziness is a side effect of Aricept and the client should therefore be advised to move slowly when rising from a sitting or lying position. Answer A is incorrect because increasing the number of pills the client takes can increase the side effects and is therefore not recommended. Answer C is incorrect because the medication should be taken at bedtime, with no regard to food. Answer D is also incorrect because bradycardia is another effect of the medication.

78. **The client has a cocaine addiction. The nurse should expect the client to be placed on which medication?**

   a. Bromocriptine (Parlodel)

   b. Disulfiram (Antabuse)

   c. Methadone

   d. THC

**Answer A is correct.** Bromocriptine (Parlodel) is classified as an anti-Parkinsonism drug and gives clients with this addiction a substitute for the neurotransmitter dopamine. It is therefore the medication utilized for addiction to cocaine.

Answer B is incorrect because Antabuse is used for alcohol abuse. Answer C is incorrect as Methadone is used for opioid addiction. Answer D is also incorrect as THC is marijuana and is not utilized for replacement therapy.

79. **A client has been placed on the drug valproic acid (Depakene). Which of the following symptoms would indicate to the nurse that the client is experiencing an adverse reaction to the drug?**

   a. Lethargy

   b. Photophobia

   c. Poor skin turgor

   d. Reported visual disturbances

**Answer A is correct.** This is because Lethargy could be an indication of hepatatoxicity. The nurse should carefully monitor for any signs of anorexia, nausea, jaundice, facial edema, vomiting, and unusual bleeding or bruising. Answers B, C, and D are incorrect as they are not clinical manifestations of adverse effects of the drug Depakene.

80. **A client with a diagnosis of Amyotrophic Lateral Sclerosis (ALS) has received a prescription riluzole (Rilutek). Which instructions should the nurse include when teaching the client about this medication? Select all that apply.**

a. Avoid any use of alcohol

b. Laboratory test will be monitored regularly

c. Medication should be taken at the same time each day

d. Report any fever to the health care provider

e. Take the medication with meals

**Answers A, B, C, and D are all correct.** A client placed on Rilutek should avoid using alcohol, report any signs of fever, and take the medication at the same time each day. These factors, along with the monitoring of laboratory values are all information that should be included in the teaching plan. Answer E is incorrect because the medication should not be taken with food.

81. **The nurse is caring for a client with leukemia who has been maintained with doxorubicin (Adriamycin). Which toxic effects of this medication should the nurse immediately report to the physician?**

a. Elevated BUN and dry, flaky skin

b. Nausea and vomiting

c. Rales and distended neck veins

d. Red discoloration of the urine

**Answer C is correct.** The medication can cause cardiotoxicity exhibited by changes in the ECG and congestive heart failure. Rales and distended neck veins are clinical manifestations of congestive heart failure and must be reported immediately. Answer A is incorrect as this effect is not specific to the medication. Answer B is incorrect because nausea and vomiting is a common side effect and therefore there is no need to report this immediately to the doctor. Answer D is incorrect because the reddish discoloration of the urine is a harmless side effect of the medication.

82. **The nurse is performing an admission history for a client recovering from a stroke. The client's dedication history reveals that the client has been taking clopidogrel (Plavix). Which clinical manifestation alerts the nurse to an adverse effect of this medication?**

   a. Epistaxis
   b. Hyperactivity
   c. Hypothermia
   d. Nausea

**Answer A is correct.** The medication Plavix is an antiplatelet and therefore epistaxis, bleeding from the nose, could indicate a severe effect. Answers B, C, and D have no direct relation to the undesired effects of the medication.

**83.** A client with angina is experiencing migraines and has received a prescription for Sumatriptan succinate (Imitrex). Which of the following nursing actions is most appropriate?

    a. Call the doctor to question the prescription order

    b. Consult social services for financial assistance with obtaining the drug

    c. Perform discharge teaching for this medication

    d. Try to obtain samples for the client to take home

**Answer A is correct.** Answer A is most appropriate in this scenario. The medication results in

cranial vasoconstriction to reduce pain, but can also cause vasoconstrictive effects. Because of this, it is contraindicated in clients who have angina. Therefore, it is necessary to contact and notify the doctor. Answer C is appropriate also, but answer A is more appropriate. Answers B and D are incorrect. These are both inappropriate actions.

**84.** A client with increased intracranial pressure is maintained on Furosemide (Lasix) and Osmitrol (Mannitol). The nurse recognizes that these two medications are administered to reverse which effect?

a. Cellular edema

b. Energy failure

c. Excessive glutamate release

d. Excessive intracellular calcium

**Answer A is correct.** The medications Lasix and Mannitol are given for their diuretic effects in decreasing cerebral edema. Answers C, B, and D are therefore incorrect.

85. **A client has an order for cisplatin (Platinol). Which medication would the nurse expect to be ordered in order to reduce renal toxicity from the cisplatin infusion?**

a. Pamidronate (Aredia)

b. Mesna (Mesenex)

c. Dexrazoxane (Zinecard)

d. Amifostine (Ethyol)

**Answer D is correct.** The drug Ethyol is used to reduce renal toxicity with cisplatin administration. Answers A, B, and C are therefore incorrect as these drugs are cytoprotectants which are not utilized for cisplatin administration.

86. **A client with a ruptured cerebral aneurysm has received an order for Nimodipine (Nimotop). Which of the following is a desired effect of this drug?**

    a. Restoration of a normal blood pressure reading

    b. Prevention of the influx of calcium into cells

    c. Prevention of the inflammatory process

    d. Dissolving of the clot that has formed

**Answer B is correct.** The medication Nimotop is a calcium channel blocker that is used to prevent calcium influx. The causation of vasospasm of the blood vessel is thought to be related to this calcium influx. Because of this, Nimotop is administered to prevent this. Answers A, C, and D are incorrect as they do not describe the action of this drug.

87. **The client with erosive gastritis has been placed on Nexium (esomeprazole). The nurse should administer the drug:**

    a. With each meal

    b. In a single dose at bedtime

    c. 30 minutes before a meal

    d. 30 minutes after meals

**Answer C is correct.** This is because Nexium is a proton

pump inhibitor that should be taken before meals. Answers A, B, and D are incorrect administration times for proton pump inhibitors like Nexium.

88. **The doctor has ordered ranitidine (Zantac) for a client with erosive gastritis. The nurse should give the medication:**

    a. 30 minutes before meals

    b. With each meal

    c. In a single dose at bedtime

    d. 60 minutes after meals

**Answer B is correct.** This is because Zantac (rantidine) is a histamine blocker that should be taken with meals for optimal effect. Note however that Tagamet (cimetidine) is a histamine blocker that can be given in one dose at bedtime. Answers A and D are incorrect as neither of these drugs should be given before or after meals.

89. **A client with gallstones and obstructive jaundice is experiencing severe itching. The doctor has ordered cholestyramine (Questran) and the client requested information as to how this medication works. Which of the following statement is the best response a nurse can give?**

a. "It binds with bile acids and is excreted in bowel movements with stool"

b. "It blocks histamine, thereby reducing the allergic response"

c. "It decreases the amount of bile in the gallbladder"

d. "It inhibits the enzyme responsible for bile excretion"

**Answer A is correct.** Questran works by binding the bile acid in the GI tract and eliminating it. This reduces the itching sensation associated with jaundice. Answers B, C, and D are incorrect as they are not answers as to how the medication works to decrease itching.

90. The nurse is looking after a client who abuses narcotics. The client is exhibiting a respiratory rate of 10 and dilated pupils. Which medication should the nurse expect to administer?

a. Chlordiazepoxide (Librium)

b. Haloperidol (Haldol)

c. Meperidine (Demerol)

d. Naloxone (Narcan)

**Answer D is correct.** The nurse should expect to administer Narcan. This is because the client is exhibiting signs of respiratory depression from the use of narcotics and therefore requires an antagonist to reverse the effects. Answer A and B are incorrect as these are antianxiety and antipsychotic medications, not narcotic-reversal drugs. Answer C is incorrect because Demerol is a narcotic that would only increase the adverse effects that the client is experiencing.

91. **The client with urinary tract infection is placed on Furadantin. He may also receive ascorbic acid. The rationale to use this additional medication is to:**

     a. Promote tissue repair
     b. Fortify mucosal repair
     c. Alkalinize the urine
     d. Acidify the urine

**Answer D is correct.** The antimicrobial activity of Furadantin is more effective in an acid urine. Because of this, ascorbic acid or vitamin C is used to acidify the urine. Answers A, B, and C are incorrect.

92. **The nurse is about to instruct client about phenytoin sodium (Dilantin). Which information would be most important to teach the client as to why the drug should not be stopped abruptly?**

The NCLEX Trainer: Pharmacology

a. A hypoglycemic reaction can develop

b. Heart block can develop

c. Status epilepticus can develop

d. The client can develop a physical dependence over time

**Answer C is correct.** A sudden discontinuation of seizure medication can cause status epilepticus to occur. This disorder is life threatening and it is therefore crucial that the client is informed about this. Answers A, B, and D are incorrect because these are not correct statements about the medication.

93. **The physician orders dopamine for a client with left ventricular failure and a high pulmonary capillary wedge pressure (PCWP) to improve ventricular function. The nurse knows that the medication is having its intended effect when:**

a. Blood pressure decreases

b. Blood pressure rises

c. Cardiac index falls

d. PCWP rises

**Answer B is correct.** The dopamine is having a desired effect when blood pressure rises. This is because it will cause vasoconstriction peripherally, but increase renal perfusion and the blood pressure will rise. Answer A is incorrect as it is the opposite of B. Answer C is also incorrect because the cardiac index will rise. Answer D is likewise incorrect because the PCWP should decrease.

94. **The physician has prescribed a Becloforte (beclomethasone) inhaler two puffs twice a day for a client with asthma. The nurse should instruct the client to report:**

    a. A sore throat
    b. Changes in mood
    c. Difficulty in sleeping
    d. Increased weight

**Answer A is correct.** This is because clients on steroid medications, including beclomethasone, can develop adverse side effects such as oral infections with candida albicans. Both a sore throat and white patches on the oral mucosa are symptoms of candida albicans and must therefore be reported immediately. Answers B, C, and D are incorrect because increased weight, difficulty sleeping, and changes in mood are all expected side effects of the medication.

95. **The nurse visits a home client with hypertension who has been maintained on a daily dose of**

methyldopa (Aldomet). The client informs the nurse that they have been experiencing symptoms of lethargy and drowsiness. The appropriate nursing intervention would be to:

a. Ask the physician to order a different antihypertensive
b. Explain to the client that these are expected side effects
c. Report the negative side effects to the physician to have the dose reduced
d. Suggest that the client take the medication at bedtime and to reevaluate next time

**Answer D is correct.** These side effects may be present with this drug but can be alleviated if the drug is taken in the evening. Taking one dose in the evening can often minimize the sedation. The nurse should nevertheless report the side effects to the physician and follow up with the client. Answers A, B, and C are incorrect.

96. The mother of a client contacts the clinic informing that nurse that her daughter cannot swallow the capsule because it is too large. The nurse finds that the medication is a capsule marked *SR*. The nurse should instruct the mother to:

a. Call the pharmacist and request an alternative preparation of the medication

b. Crush the medication and administer it with 8 oz. of liquid

c. Open the capsule and mix the medication with ice cream

d. Stop the medication and inform the physician at the follow-up visit

**Answer A is correct.** *SR* stands for sustained release and these medications cannot be altered. The mother should therefore be instructed to request an alternative preparation of the medication from the pharmacist. Answers B and C are incorrect because crushing or opening the capsule is not allowed. Answer D is also incorrect as it is not necessary to notify the doctor immediately.

97. **The client with rheumatoid arthritis has been placed on aspirin gr. xx TID and prednisone 10 mg BID for 2 years. The most important assessment the nurse should make is whether the client has experienced:**

a. Blurred vision

b. A decreased sense of appetite

c. Headaches

d. Tarry stools

**Answer D is correct.** This is because aspirin impedes clotting by blocking prosta-glandin synthesis. This can lead to bleeding. A common side effect of the medication

Prednisone is gastric irritation, which can likewise lead to bleeding. Tarry stools indicate bleeding in the upper GI system which should be immediately reported. Answers A, B, and D are incorrect. Although these should also be noted and reported, they are not the most important assessment for the nurse to make and are therefore incorrect.

98. **A client scheduled for disc surgery informs the nurse that she frequently uses the herbal supplement kava-kava (piper methysticum). The nurse should immediately report this to the doctor because kava-kava:**

    a. Depresses the immune system, so infection is more of a problem

    b. Eliminates the need for antimicrobial therapy following surgery

    c. Increases the effects of anesthesia and post-operative analgesia

    d. Increases urinary output, so a urinary catheter will be needed post-operatively

**Answer C is correct.** The herbal kava-kava can increase the effects of anesthesia and post-operative analgesia. Answers A, B, and D are incorrect because they are not related to the use of kava-kava.

99. The physician has ordered several medications including Beta Blocker Atenolol for a client with Congestive Heart Failure. The client requested information as to how this medication works. Which of the following statement is the best response a nurse can give?

    a. "It causes vasodilation of coronary vessels"

    b. "It increases the heart rate and forces contraction"

    c. "It decreases the heart rate and forces contraction"

    d. "It reduces myocardial oxygen demands"

**Answer C is correct.** Beta blockers decrease the heart rate and force contraction, thereby reducing vasoconstriction by antagonizing Beta receptors in the myocardium and vasculature. Answers A and D are incorrect as they refer to the action of nitrates and Calcium Channel Blockers such as Diltiazem. Answer B is also incorrect because it is the opposite of Answer C and therefore untrue.

100. A client with a detached retina has just been admitted and surgery has been scheduled. The nurse knows that the pre-op ophthalmic medication most likely to be ordered for the client will be:

    a. Atropine sulfate

    b. Carbamylcholine

c. Pilocarpine

d. Timolol maleate

**Answer A is correct.** This is because the medications used pre-op to widely dilate the pupil are Mydriatic drugs. Both Atropine sulfate and Epinephrine HCI are commonly used. Answer B and C are incorrect because these are miotics used for certain types of lens implants and glaucoma. Answer D is also incorrect because Timolol maleate is a beta blocker used for glaucoma.

101. **A client is about to be discharged with an order for bishydroxycoumarin (Dicumarol). Which instructions should be included in the teaching plan?**

  a. The client should shave with an electric razor

  b. The client should take the medication prior to eating

  c. It is for the physician to teach the client about the medication

  d. If the client misses a doe, he should take a double dose next time

**Answer A is correct.** The medication Dicumarol is an anticoagulant drug and because of this, one of the dangers is bleeding. Using a safetly razor can lead to bleeding through cuts and the client should therefore use an electric razor.

Answer B is incorrect because although the drug should be taken at the same time every day, there is no relation to meals. Answer C is incorrect and Answer D is also incorrect because, due to the danger of bleeding, missed doses should not be made up.

# Section 4: Study and Exam Preparation Tips

Studying for the NCLEX is a daunting challenge for every nursing student. Despite this, it is completely manageable and with the right approach, and success can be guaranteed.

In preparing for the NCLEX, there are three central elements that are of most important: **understanding, organisation, and practice.** This study guide is designed for those who already have a good understanding of nursing practice. *Section 2* of the guide is simply designed to refresh your memory and help you retain essential information that you will need to answer the practice questions in *Section 3.*

In this section, we have compiled some essential review strategies that will assist you in effective preparation for the NCLEX!

## Study Tips:

- **Learning the details comes first!**
- -Before going through the questions, it is important that you have come to grasp with the content that is being tested.
- -Practice questions are designed to test and further your knowledge, and to make sure you know how to

answer the questions efficiently and successfully.

- **Repetition is key!**

-Memorizing is key when it comes to dealing with conversion factors, laboratory values, among other things. It is therefore useful to devote a set time each day to studying the information.

-On top of this, we encourage you to make best use of the time you spend commuting by continually going over key points.

-Repeating information just before you go to sleep also helps you memorize information you find particularly difficult to retain.

- **Test yourself!**

-As the old saying goes, practice is the key to success. The questions presented in this guide are representative of what you should expect in the NCLEX exam.

-Testing yourself is essential to knowing whether you are well prepared for the exam.

-Make sure to practice as much as possible and once you are getting closer to the  actual exam, time yourself, allowing approximately one minute per question.

- **Learn from your mistakes!**

-If there are questions you haven't answered correctly, then see whether you understand the rationale and go over your revision notes again to make sure you have understood it fully.

-Make sure to test yourself again on questions that you initially answered incorrectly.

-All questions in this guide are numbered. Make sure to note down the questions you answered incorrectly and skip forward to these questions next time!

## Exam Tips:

These are tips you should apply when you are sitting the exam. Try to also apply these when you are going over practice questions so it becomes second nature!

- **Read the questions carefully!**
-Being alert is key to successfully passing the NCLEX! Skimming through questions is the mistake most often made.
-It is crucial to make sure you read the question carefully and that you fully understand what it is the question is asking.
-If necessary, reword the question in your own words. This often helps in crafting an appropriate answer.

- **Look for keywords!**
-Keywords will help you work through the questions more efficiently.
-It is also advisable to avoid answers that include keywords such as all, always, every, except, must, never, no, none and only because they are rarely correct as they often limit or qualify the actual correct answer.

- **Use the method of elimination!**
-This is particularly useful if you are not straight away sure which option is the correct answer.
-Eliminate the answers that are clearly wrong, incorrect, or appear unfit until you cannot eliminate anymore.

-Another tip here is to look out for vague answers. Avoid vague answers and if you spot one, eliminate it!

- **The true-false test.**
-Treat each option as a true-false question and choose the option that is the 'most true'.

- **Trust your common sense!**
-Even if you're not 100% sure, knowing that you have studied rigorously and have gained a good knowledge of the content, it is often better to trust your instinct rather than risk running out of time.
-Even more than instinct, try and use your common sense and re-read the question again to see whether there is a key aspect you have overlooked at first sight!
-Another strategy that you can use is to read the question, answer the question and pick the option that most closely matches your answer.

- **Look for similar options.**
-Looking for the odd answer is a test strategy that can also prove very useful. See whether the three similar options are related to a completely different topic and use the method of elimination or/and the true-false test to narrow down your correct answer.

- **Look for opposite/echo options.**
-If two questions are the opposite of one another, chances are that one of them is correct.

# Section 5: Final Notes

I'd like to take this opportunity to thank you for downloading this book. I hope you now have a solid foundation, and that this guide has helped you equip yourself with the knowledge to achieving success with the NCLEX Exam!

My final piece of advice - no matter how diligent you are in your studies, your best learning will come from proactively practicing questions over and over again. I recommend revisiting the questions you have found difficult to constantly refresh and build on your knowledge as you progress.

I sincerely wish you the best of luck in your exam.

Best wishes,

Eva Regan

Made in the USA
Lexington, KY
02 April 2016